CANCER

A CIRCLE OF SEASONS

A way to journal and pray
through life's challenges

First published in 2017 by Columba Press
23 Merrion Square North, Dublin 2
www.columba.ie

ISBN: 978-1-78218-318-1

Set in Tisa Pro 10/15

Cover design by Alba Esteban | Columba Press

Book design by Helene Pertl & Alba Esteban

Printed by Jellyfish Solutions

CANCER

A CIRCLE OF SEASONS

A way to journal and pray
through life's challenges

Anne Alcock

COLUMBA PRESS

DUBLIN

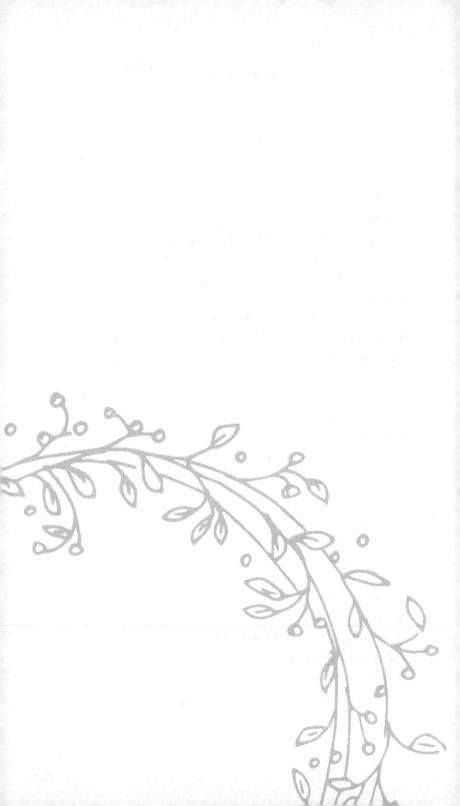

CONTENTS

Dedicated to those involved in cancer research: oncologists, surgeons, radiographers, nurses, ancillary staff, and those engaged in follow-up services

May the Lord
bless and protect you,
May the Lord's face
radiate with joy because of you.
May He be gracious to you,
show you His favour
and give you His peace.

Numbers 6:24–26

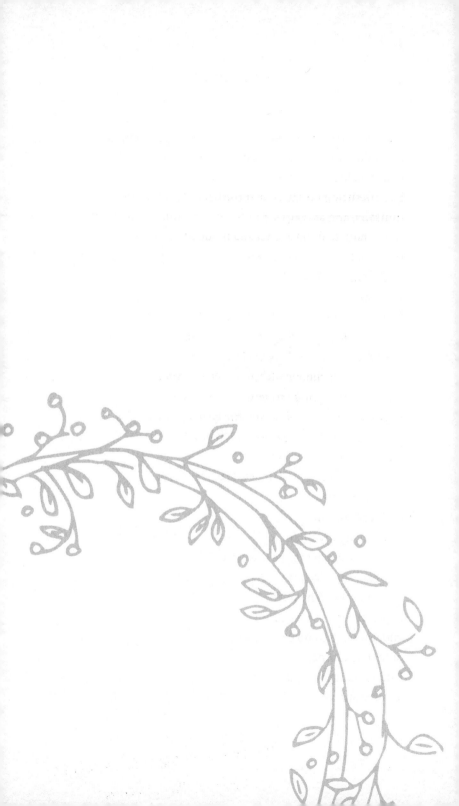

PREFACE

I have had this inner sense that something is going on,
or is about to happen, or that I have to do.
I have no idea what it is.
So I am sitting on the side of the bed,
thinking, and asking God,
'What best attitude can I bring to my life?
How am I supposed to live it?'
And suddenly, I clearly *see* a word.
The word is 'YES'.
I say aloud, 'Yes'.
'That's it? Just 'yes'?'
Actually it feels like a perfect fit.
A comfortable knowledge,
one that I recognise already.
A 'yes' to whatever is coming up in my future.
A 'yes' to my life.
But, being me, I would love
to have that word
somehow affirmed.
(Before I commit!)
So I pick up my Bible.
Do I really expect to see the word, 'yes'?
My head says 'No way.'
My soul says 'Why not?'
I open the Bible at random.
and, there, with no page-turning
or text-scanning,
I am looking straight down
at the word 'yes'.

It occurs at the beginning
of what looks like
an expansive, welcoming invitation –

'Yes, eat and drink,
lover and beloved, drink deeply.'
Song of Songs 5:1

Co-incidence, or God-incidence?
Either way, it is my experience.
I feel calm, affirmed, open.
It's a 'yes' from me
to whatever it is,
I am saying 'yes' to.
It turns out to be a cancer diagnosis,
but ...
... so much more.
An inner pilgrimage,
a venture into the unknown.
Cancer treatment
is no longer a secret
or an uncommon journey;
inevitably,
it is a unique one
for each of us who embarks on it.
A special 'aloneness' is ours,
even within family, friends and loving supports.
For me, single (and content to be),
this venture with God
became an Adventure.

Adventure: an undertaking involving uncertainty and risk. (Encarta)
Etymology, Latin *adventus*, p.p. of *advenire* – to arrive. (Webster)

PSALM 139

O Lord you have examined my heart
and know everything about me.
You know when I sit or stand.
When far away, you know my every thought.
You chart the path ahead of me
and tell me where to stop and rest.
You know what I am going to say, before I even say it.
You both precede and follow me,
and lay your hand of blessing on my head.
This is too glorious, too wonderful to believe!
If I go up to heaven, you are there.
If I go down to the place of the dead, you are there.
If I ride the morning winds to the farthest oceans,
Your hand will guide me – your strength will support me.
If I try to hide in the darkness, the night becomes light
around me. For even darkness cannot hide from God.
To you the night shines as bright as day.
Darkness and light are both alike to you.
You made all the delicate inner parts of my body and
knit them together in my mother's womb. Thank you for
making me so wonderfully complex. It is amazing to think
about ... You saw me before I was born, and scheduled each
day of my life, before I began to breathe ...
How precious it is Lord, to realise that you are thinking
about me constantly. I can't even count how many times
a day your thoughts are turned towards me, and when I
wake in the morning, you are still thinking of me.

– Living Bible

SPRING

Walk in wisdom, redeeming the time.

Colossians 4:5 NKV

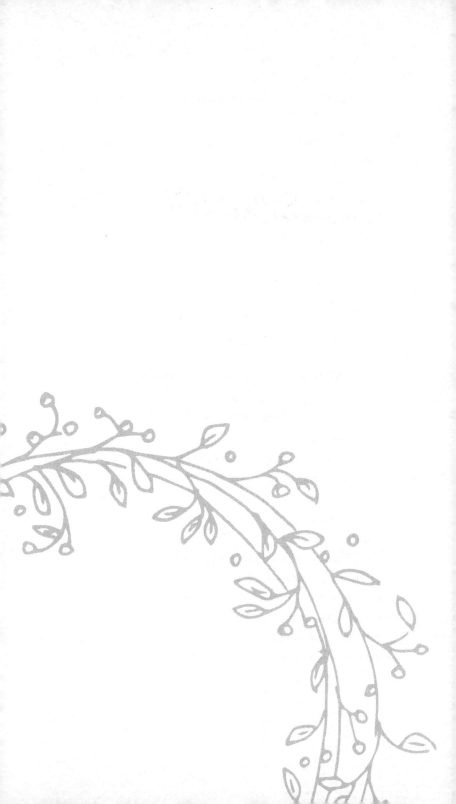

1

I NOTICE SOMETHING DIFFERENT

My bra is getting to me.
I am wriggling with discomfort.
Finding that loosening the band,
or adjusting the cup,
isn't changing things.
There is a sharp jab on my right side,
going on for some days now
like a burning, under my breast.
But it is early Spring,
I've had a little break, relaxing, walking, eating,
of course I must have 'put on' a bit,
so no longer fit my bra.
Surely?
Yet the stinging pain is distracting me.
That bra has to come off,
and straight away I see
the bright red band marks under my breast,
very inflamed on the right side
– and an obvious lump.
Then I remember
that weeks ago
I did notice a 'dent' under my right breast,
which wasn't under the left one.
A dent? Like a thumb had pressed deep under a rib.
Didn't look like dimpling.
So I noticed one dent,
and dismissed it. Easy.

PRAYING
Attentive awareness

Lord,
I too easily dismiss
what I don't want to notice.
Look away. Forget about it.
Don't disturb the peace.
'I'm fine.'
There are plenty of interesting distractions
and necessities
that need my attention.
After that, I'll see.
But for now,
I prefer not to know...
Is this my 'ostrich-in-the-sand' approach
when my body knows something
and is trying to tell me?
What strange idea do I hold
That makes me believe I can't get sick ?
That this 'attribute' belongs to others?
I need to think about this.
When I am ready, help me to risk
bringing to awareness
what I would prefer to step away from.

....

Just one word or sentence might be the one that opens the way for your own journey, inwards and onwards.

- My life today in a paragraph:

- Something that is looking for attention at the moment:

- The letter you write to yourself about this, says:

- Your favourite distractions/avoidances/rationalisations are:

- 'Resolutions are just for New Year and last three days max.' Discuss.

- Five keywords for journaling:

Prayer-starter
- Write a note to the Lord, about anything on your mind, and sign it. Then, with soft shoulders, and relaxed jaw, sit gently with the words 'Be still and know, that I am God.' allowing their meaning to settle in.

- Insights from prayer:

The Lord waits to be gracious to you.

Isaiah 30:18

2

SEEING THE G.P.

I decide to see my doctor,
but no rush.
Things have settled down.
The wired bra is off, the sports top is on,
and the redness has gone.
However it is the occasional pulling and tweaking
from near, or within, the now much paler lump
that makes me phone for an appointment.
'Oh, just a general check-up.
Friday week will do.'
Friday week comes, I am called in,
and truthfully I can say
'Never better!' when asked.
...'except that I found a lump.'
Palpating the area, my doctor confirms this.
'Yes. You have a lump. Very hard, isn't it?'
We look at each other.
He makes the face I am probably making too,
and sets up a referral.
How do I feel? I feel suspended but calm.
Like facing an inevitability,
also expectant, curious,
in a knowing kind of way.
And now begins the first day
of probably many days of 'wait-ings'.

PRAYING
Waiting

Lord,
Show me how to wait well.
To keep my mind steady and grounded
in today.
Not tomorrow.
Or next week.
Or next year.
Thank you for the practice
I have had over the last years
in learning to wait,
while caring for my mother.
To wait on administration
and forms and departmental letters
and phone-calls.
Learning to let the wheels turn
hands loose, and allow things to be –
without trying to fill a space
which is actually meant
for something else,
at another time.

JOURNAL
For you

. . . .

Just one word or sentence might be the one that opens the way for your own journey, inwards and onwards.

- At the moment, 'waiting' is about:

- The emotions/thoughts that waiting brings up, are:

- Your supports during 'waiting times':

- 'What's especially difficult about waiting is …'
  Finish the sentence and write onwards.

- Memories of waiting for, waiting in, waiting on:

- Five keywords for journaling:

Prayer-starter
- Lifting shoulders to your ears, with straight arms, clench your fists for a moment or two. Relax on an outbreath. Repeat. Now with hands relaxed in your lap, bring your attention, body, mind and spirit, to the present moment and God's presence in the Now. 'Now' is what you have, where you are.

- Insights from prayer:

Let me hear what the Lord will speak,
for he will speak peace...

Psalm 85:8 NRSV

3
FIRST CONSULTATION

I am on my way to the hospital.
I didn't sleep well last night.
Nerves. I think this lump could be malignant.
Or at least it is something that should not be there.
Fingers crossed. I feel a bit sick.
I don't have a car, and the bus
seems to be crawling through the morning traffic,
dropping me at the hospital just three minutes
before the appointment time.
I was tense anyway, but now I am on high alert,
noticing details – the chairs are wipe-clean comfortable,
there is a water cooler in the corner,
the radio is chattering away – like my mind.
There is no way and nowhere to hide.
Yes, that is my name, loud and clear.
I am escorted to the consulting room.
Lying on the examination couch,
arms above head.
I sense I am in a safe pair of hands.
These fingers are very experienced.
A preliminary assessment, and then
'Is there anything you want to ask me?'
Her calm tone infers that there is all the time in the world.
I am hugely reassured, and have only to speak, and yet my
mouth is suddenly dry, and it is in a husky whisper, unable
to swallow, that I reply,
'I don't know what to ask.'

PRAYING

Lord, when the words run out
and any thoughts
have disappeared
over the horizon,
there is nothing to say any more,
nothing to know.
All I can do,
is stay with what 'is',
acknowledging
where I am,
how I am,
how that feels.
I can rest in silence
and let your Presence surround me.

Just one word or sentence might be the one that opens the way for your own journey, inwards and onwards.

- 'I don't know what to ask ...'
  Finish the sentence and write onwards as your story.

- Five things you want information about ... because:

- A reassuring conversation with a 'tensed-up' part of you:

- 'Relaxing' happens when:

- Five keywords for journaling:

Prayer-starter
- Become aware of your breathing, and without effort, allow it to become deeper, by relaxing your shoulders and jaw. Choose a calming prayer – mantra – and repeat it for a while on your outbreath.

- Insights from prayer:

Let your steadfast love, O Lord,
be upon us, even as we hope in you.

Psalm 33:22

4

THE MAMMOGRAM SQUEEZE

I once tried to describe the
'Mammogram Experience' to a friend.
He visibly winced.
This is a most appropriate response,
no matter how useful and valuable
and necessary the procedure.
Today I am in the cheerful care of two nurses,
who put me into a cotton gown,
and have a good laugh
when they hear that my only allergy is wine.
'How unfortunate!' says one,
while the other stands me
close against a shiny, white mammogram machine
and manoeuvres me into the most unlikely positions;
arms clasping the machine, shoulders down,
bum out, hips turned sideways,
legs placed like a sprinter on the blocks.
Then, truthfully,
'This will be a little bit of a squeeze ...'
and I take a sharp intake of breath,
as scooped-up flesh squashes
between a flat 'plate' and a 'paddle.'
(Who makes these names up?)
But immediately
that brief pressure eases,
and the release is instant.
I breathe out.
It's okay. It's manageable.
And those nurses were the best.

PRAYING

Lord,
I joke,
I flinch,
I laugh again,
'making light.'
But under all that,
I hold this large,
upright machine with its x-raying eyes
in huge respect.
What it sees,
will set my path!
This is such a big thought,
that it seems best
to take it lightly,
because until we know something
'for sure'
we don't know
anything.

Just one word or sentence might be the one that opens the way for your own journey, inwards and onwards.

· When out of your comfort-zone, you:

· 'My ways of handling surprises or the unexpected, are ...' Finish the sentence and write onwards.

· 'Uncertainty reminds me of ...'
  Finish the sentence and write onwards.

· Best coping skills, learned when:

· Best relaxation techniques:

· Five keywords for journaling:

Prayer-starter
· Reading and reflecting on any verse or verses that 'speak to you' from Psalm 40.

· Insights from prayer:

When I look at your heavens,
the work of your fingers,
the moon and stars that you have established;
what are human beings that you are mindful of them,
mortals that you care for them?

Psalm 8:3–4 NRSV

5

ULTRASOUND AND MORE

I am transported into a world of consoles,
transducers and gels
and awesome, incomprehensible technology.
This is ultrasound territory.
Flat on my back and in a blue gown,
I get a sideways glimpse
of my breast's measured and incomprehensible secrets –
on screen. I am reminded
of compass-markings, which
I equally don't understand.
Inaudible pulses convert into images,
and I am fascinated
by the explanations and the expertise.
Then soft wads of paper
wipe down gel-sticky skin
and my right breast prepares itself
for it's core-biopsy moment.
A topical anaesthetic numbs the skin,
and a nurse stands quietly poised,
with a small dressing,
ready for when,
with a decisive click, the biopsy needle
painlessly bites out its allotted portion of tissue.

PRAYING
The wonders of creation and of science

Lord,
I am struck by a sense of awe.
Not only at the technology,
the science and the expertise
but also by an awe which moves me
to both deep gratitude, and
a sense of humbleness.
(Humility sounds too remote.
It is humbleness.)
These tests and checks
available to me –
May I never take this for granted.
May I live worthy of it.

....

Just one word or sentence might be the one that opens the way for your own journey, inwards and onwards.

- The part of created or scientific life that especially interests you is:

- 'My own life-story began when ...'
  Write onwards.

- The gifts you inherited, and the talents you've discovered:

- A psalm of thanksgiving for your being, and life thus far:

- Five keywords for journaling:

Prayer-starter
- Gaze at stars, night skies, dawn or sunset, and/or reflect on Psalm 8.

- Insights from prayer:

But as for me, I know that my redeemer lives and that He will stand upon the earth at last. And I know that...this body shall see God.

Job 19:26

6

LIVING WITH DYING

Today I visited an undertakers,
in a spirit of enquiry –
rather like shopping –
and raised the sort of questions
I have only ever asked
about someone else.
How much for a grave plot?
How much for a coffin?
Wicker, wood, or willow?
What about organ donation?
Or is mine a whole-body donation
organised through an Anatomical Gift Programme?
Well, I made my choice
for that interface between two worlds,
perhaps 'before time',
but precisely to allow time
to live well for the remainder
of my time,
in this world.
As Carl Jung said,
'You cannot live well, unless you can die well.'

PRAYING
My death as part of my life

Lord, let me live well,
through accepting death.
as a fact of life
as and when it will come.
I don't mean to anticipate,
I don't mean to 'dwell'
and no-one is talking about death.
But one day I will die, so let me
take this as an opportunity,
however far ahead,
to acknowledge, accept,
and do whatever is needed
while I can do so,
in a spirit of pragmatic peace.

Just one word or sentence might be the one that opens the way for your own journey, inwards and onwards.

· 'If you can die well, you can live well' (Jung)
  To me, this means:

· 'My image of life after death is …'
  Finish the sentence and write onward.

· The effect on your life as lived now.

· The practical arrangements that are in place for your own death, are:

· Someone once said, 'I am not afraid of dying. I am only afraid of dying with regrets.' You?

· Five keywords for journaling:

Prayer-starter
· Read the Gospel of John, chapter 14, slowly, putting your name at every full stop. Stay where you find yourself found by the Lord.

· Insights from prayer:

O Lord ... you know everything about me.
You know when I sit or stand ...
You know what I am going to say, before I even say it.
You both precede and follow me,
and place your hand of blessing on my head.

Psalm 139:1,3,5. Living Bible

7

OUT OF SORTS

Yesterday I missed a call.
(Perhaps it is about an appointment?)
I ring the number back. No reply.
I ring again today.
They haven't heard of me. They can't find me?
I am given another number to try.
I leave a message. Get a call back.
My appointment 'isn't yet in the system'.
What does this mean? What 'system'?
Your appointment will be made shortly, and as soon as it is,
you will be getting a call. Is that okay?'
'Yes,' I say, grudgingly, 'I guess.'
Mine is a most ungracious reply.
I'm feeling (inaccurately)
that all power
to manage my own life
is slipping away.
I am insecure, and certainly over-reacting when I say,
urgently, 'Will you be sure to text me as soon as you know?'
There is practised patience on the other side, and later on
I get both a call and a text.
Everything perfectly sorted.
Irrationally, even this irritates me
because now I don't want to be smothered by care.
When I began this, I wanted to be found.
Now I don't know what I want.

PRAYING
The whole me

Lord,
It doesn't have to 'make sense'.
It is fine to be 'all over the place'.
(I nearly added 'every now and then',
which just proves I am not sure
I really believe that it is fine).
So now I pray that others can bear with me
while I behave like a bag of cats at times,
and feel like a pouty baby at others.
It's all out of the same pot.
And the rest is in there somewhere too.

. . . .

Just one word or sentence might be the one that opens the way for your own journey, inwards and onwards.

· 'What particularly irritates me is ...'
  Finish the sentence and write onwards.

· Pro-active, passive, or passive-aggressive when frustrated? Who would tell you?

· 'The roles I play when out of sorts ...'
  Finish the sentence and write onwards.

· A dialogue between yourself and one of the roles:

· Proven techniques for restoring harmony:

· Five keywords for journaling:

Prayer-starter
· Bring the frustrated part of you into a prayer-place where you visualise the presence of Jesus, Mary, or a saint or an angel or other Wisdom figure. Use 'I' (I feel) statements, rather than 'they' (blame) accusations, and then become quiet. Stay, heart open, and listen.

· Insights from prayer:

Be beautiful in your hearts.

1 Peter 3:4

8

'OH, I CAN MANAGE!'

'The best gift you can receive, is time.'
I read that somewhere. It is worth reflecting on,
and right now I am receiving this gift, from friends.
For an 'I'm totally fine, I can manage' kind of person,
this is mind and heart stretching.
I am due at the hospital for test results and the day starts
with a text from the lads nearby,
'Thinking of you. We have everything crossed!'
Then the gift of generosity:
'If there is anything we can do, just say.'
'I won't be around for a while', texts another friend,
'but can I give you a hand this week? You only need to ask.'
That's the rub; actually asking.
I haven't told that many people, but those who know
are personifying what friendship means.
'Part of service, is to allow others to serve us.'
I read that too, once, but again
it didn't register, and I couldn't apply it to myself
– I shrank from either pride, or a false humility.
But of course it applies to me, exactly as to anyone else,
So I begin to text, asking to meet
after my appointment. Then, remembering that she
has a lot on today, I briefly waver and assure her,
truthfully, that it is 'fine' if she is too busy.
Equally predictable, she texts back the three words
which say it all – about friendship – 'I'll be there.'

PRAYING
Being a friend, receiving friendship

Lord,
You know that life has made me 'independent'.
I am not used to being 'carried'
and I know I would struggle
if it felt confining.
But it feels spacious –
as well as supportive.
Like being encouraged to
drop into the well-used roominess of
a capacious carrier bag.
My life, alongside a lot of others'
– equally precious.

Just one word or sentence might be the one that opens the way for your own journey, inwards and onwards.

- 'Me and my friends ...'
  Continue.

- The best 'gift' of friendship ever received:

- 'As a friend I ...'
  Finish the sentence and write onward.

- 'Life is all of a piece and you are part of it.'
  Your response.

- Five keywords for journaling:

Prayer-starter
- Remembering the first person who really touched your heart. Thinking of special friends and wishing/sending them love and strength or other quality, in the Lord.

- Insights from prayer:

Bless the Lord, O my soul,
and all that is within me,
Bless his holy name.
Bless the Lord, O my soul,
and do not forget all his benefits.

Psalm 103:1–2 NRSV

9

DIAGNOSIS DAY

I am early, so I wander into the nearby church.
It is warm and quiet.
There won't be a big surprise about today's diagnosis.
The strange little tweaks and jabs in my right breast
are saying something loud and clear.
Once in the clinic, all is quiet. I drink some cold water from
the dispenser, and my eyes follow the staff padding to and
fro, until I am taken into the consulting room.
The surgeon has my file, and with a steady gaze, she says
the words that she must say many times every week.
'Well, its cancer,' she says.
With a thud of stunning truth in my chest, I feel instantly
conveyed into a huge human sisterhood.
So it is breast cancer.
There was no beating about the bush. I like that.
Treatment and tests will follow,
the surgical options proposed.
Finally, I am given a positive recommendation
for the meantime. 'Don't go and change anything;
exercise, live your life, and don't go and diet!
People go and start juicing and all sorts of things,
and they just get weak, and don't heal.'
Tweaking those healthy recommendations ever so slightly,
I meet a friend and we indulge in some guilt-free carrot
cake, with cream-cheese topping, in a garden centre. I buy
some plants, and a little ceramic duck for my garden. I
realise later this is a sitting duck. Gulp!

PRAYING

Lord,
Life hasn't been stopped
by the word 'cancer'.
Life has changed,
and with your help
I can 'live change'.
Let me take it
day by day in balance,
as it is given.
And thank you today,
for facts,
for sound advice,
and for the sensitivity of a friend
who realised the healthiness
of balancing a visit to a hospital
with a visit to a garden centre.
A place of growth and life.

....

Just one word or sentence might be the one that opens the way for your own journey, inwards and onwards.

- A fact of life you are dealing with at the moment:

- 'Positive recommendations for living well, are ...'
  Finish the sentence and write onwards.

- Practical life-changes include:

- How can you best 'live change':

- 'My life-balance list would look like ...'
  Finish the sentence and write onwards.

- Five keywords for journaling:

Prayer-starter
- Engage in some way with nature – aware of yourself as created moment by moment, from birth to death, and into eternal life. Invite your Creator to help you live well, in peace, each moment as it is given. 'Let me abide in your tent forever, find refuge under the shelter of your wings ...' Psalm 61:4

- Insights from prayer:

In quietness and in trust shall be your strength.

Isaiah 30:15

10

CLEARING MY MIND

I am 'keeping occupied'.
But not frantic.
In fact, I feel strangely serene
and perhaps I am numb
as I wait for tests.
There are no Amazing Projects
but between work,
and, as recommended,
'continuing to live' my life
I am culling and clearing.
Clothes, cupboards, books,
all sorted, sifted and bagged,
and finally, healingly, disposed of.
Bringing a conscious calming,
a focused mindfulness,
a widened mental space,
a deeper praying place,
and a clearer, tidy, physical space.
'Tidy car, tidy mind,' a taxi driver once told me.
Well, I've no car but it's a proven truth,
'Tidy house, tidier mind.'

PRAYING

Lord,
All 'preparation'
is actually in the dark.
How can we ever know what's ahead?
But clearing out,
and tidying up,
has tidied my mind
and calmed my heart
as I wait,
swinging gently,
between fewer thoughts
in this in-between space.

JOURNAL
For you

··

Just one word or sentence might be the one that opens the way for your own journey, inwards and onwards.

· 'Blocked' or 'stuck' refers to:

· Your best way of coping at the moment?

· 'Nothing can change!'
  Write a two-way dialogue with the speaker.

· A de-cluttering programme would include:

· 'The positive actions I can take, are ...'
  Finish the sentence as a list.

· Five keywords for journaling:

Prayer-starter
· Act on anything above that you need to, and then pray from a clearer mental space, perhaps choosing a short repetitive prayer phrase (mantra).

· Insights from Prayer:

Be kind to one another, tender-hearted, forgiving one another, just as God has forgiven you.

Ephesians 4:32

11

FORGIVING TODAY

What does it take to forgive?
It doesn't have to take actual
or potential illness, or cancer,
to coax forgiveness out of its inner cave
(Although certainly, I'm finding that it helps).
The priorities change.
What mattered before
no longer matters now.
Why drag along forever
what is not needful?
Just a habit.
What about forgiving *now*
instead of 'when ...'?
Who is supposed to change?
Do I dare to loosen my grip,
stretch my shut-down heart and tight-balled fist,
offering instead an easy 'You're welcome' to everyone
and especially to a someone,
without prejudice,
without reserve?
I am glad for the other night's dream
where I kissed and forgave from the past.
'You've returned to the real X,' I said, and felt tender.

PRAYING

Lord this time is precious.
It is like I am sifting the gold out of the trash.
Letting go of what isn't significant
Including those residual hurts,
resentments
and self-righteous angers.
With your help,
I surrender to an act of truth and openness,
a commitment to inner hospitality.
Gratefully, I accept your example
and your offer of freedom.

....

Just one word or sentence might be the one that opens the way for your own journey, inwards and onwards.

· 'Forgiveness for me is about ...'
  Finish the sentence and write onwards.

· 'Don't ask me to forgive.'
  Write a dialogue as, or with, the speaker.

· Your own experience of being forgiven:

· Remembered stories, inspirations or examples of forgiveness:

· Five keywords for journaling:

Prayer-starter
· In the presence of the Lord, acknowledge what is true within yourself around forgiveness or un-forgiveness and where you are with that. Accept struggle within your own heart as normal. Pray even from within conflict. Be patient with yourself.

· Insights from prayer:

I have calmed and quieted my soul
like a weaned child with its mother;
my soul is like the weaned child that is with me.

Psalm 131:2 NRSV

12

MRI SYMPHONY

I am about to be MRI-ed.

In the changing cubicle, I am handed the blue gown. I slip into it, with confident familiarity.

But, … 'er, other way round, Anne!'

A canula with line is inserted into my arm 'for the dye'. Soon I am lying face-down on what looks like a large massage-couch positioned in front of a giant bagel. Noise-reducing earphones are placed over my ears, and a tubed bulb is pressed into my palm 'For emergencies!'.

'What would an 'emergency' look like?'

'Oh anything! You might feel unwell or something. Off you go!'

I have the sensation of being slid backwards into a tunnel and then halting. I must stay completely still. The only thing I am aware of is my breath. It feels quite jagged, so I consciously slow it down with a mantra. Then I begin to hear sounds, and I get the point of the earphones.

There are loud thuds counterpointed with lighter taps and clicks. A bizarre symphony.

I pretend I am listening to an orchestra. From time to time, the nurses' voices break through, encouraging. 'Good GIRL, Anne, Good GIRL!' Now I know what a pet dog feels like. Nice. I feel lulled into a paradoxical comfort zone. The machine gives a last loud clack, and falls silent.

I am whooshed out. The line in my arm is removed and suddenly two nurses are pressing firmly with gauze and speaking quickly 'Close your elbow!' Blood is squirting in a miniature arc onto the floor. They start mopping. 'Keep your elbow very tight. You're a Bleeder!'

PRAYING

Lord, today I inadvertently became a child again.
I didn't know how to put a gown on.
I needed an explanation of 'Emergency'.
I pretended that I was listening to an MRI orchestra,
I learned how it feels to be a soothed pet,
And I experienced again a child's comfort, when blood is
spurting and someone else knows what to do,
so everything is okay.

JOURNAL
For you

....

Just one word or sentence might be the one that opens the way for your own journey, inwards and onwards.

· Favourite music to listen to:

· The positive sounds and smells from childhood are:

· 'The times I felt "taken care of" as a child were ...'
  Finish the sentence and write onwards.

· 'The places where we played were ...'
  Finish the sentence and write onward.

· Your 'inner child' comes to life again (joyful, comforted, needy, fretful, playful, etc.). How do you respond?

· Take a walk with your 'inner child.'
  Write the conversation you have.

· Five keywords for journaling:

Prayer-starter
· Enjoy doing something childlike (as distinct from childish). Gaze, touch, taste, and experience nature and beauty with a child's senses. Play, pray.

· Insights from prayer:

Go to the land that I will show you.

Gen 12:1

13

ALL CHANGE!

'This is what is called an adventure.'
These words energise me.
It was a woman speaking to her child,
years ago, a rail strike coincided with a dustbin-strike
and everyone stood stranded in Waterloo station with
luggage and rubbish all around.
This is what is called an adventure?
Am I embarking on my own kind of adventure?
The MRI test is back. All change.
A different adventure.
The tumour site is 'awkward',
so surgery is not an option at the moment.
The tumour must first be shrunk;
so, chemotherapy.
Life will change for some time.
That is the new story.
'It is not good news,
but it's a journey,
and you just go through with it,
and you come out the other end.'
Well, I choose to embark on this journey
as my own adventure.
Amen.

PRAYING

Lord,
I reach out and take your Hand
to guide me through
a place I have never been before.
It isn't uncharted territory, and
I expect to meet others on the way.
But each of us has their own path,
and I am asking to set off on mine
with curiosity, optimism, and openness.

JOURNAL
For you

. . . .

Just one word or sentence might be the one that opens the way for your own journey, inwards and onwards.

· Your inner/outer journey at the moment:

· You feel:

· Plans that have been disrupted, or put on hold are:

· Imaging this in a creative form (colour, fabric, foliage, wood, clay. etc.):

· 'What I really need to trust at the moment is ...' Finish the sentence and write onwards.

· If you had one word to sum up this time, it would be ...? Expand on this.

· Five keywords for journaling:

Prayer-starter
· 'Where are you, God, in this?' Asked in hope and with the expectation, that 'where' will be revealed.

· Insights from prayer:

SUMMER

Before you call I will answer, and while you are still
speaking, I will hear.

Isaiah 65:24

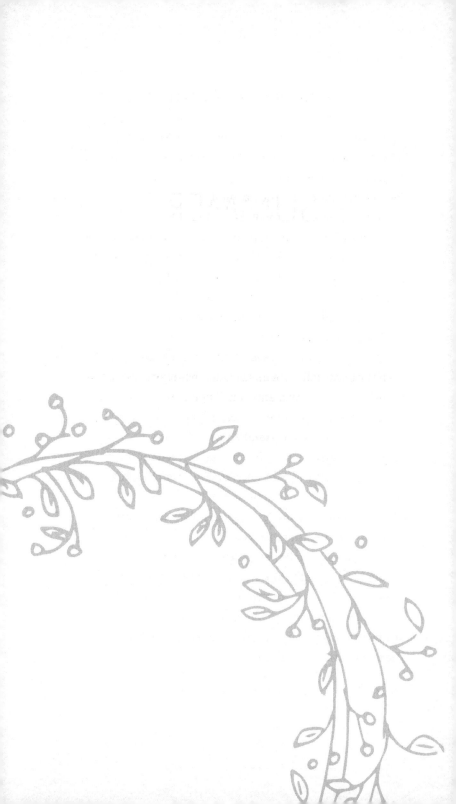

14

ONCOLOGY APPOINTMENT

I spend the morning of my first chemo consultancy
in my tiny garden, stringing cherry tomatoes and creating
supports for eager runner beans.
Then I catch the bus to the hospital.
It is hot and very bright today
and looking beyond the bulk of a sweating man beside me,
I notice for the first time, the intense Summer-green of the
glossy-leaved bushes along the road. So full of life!
I trust that I am too, when, in the hospital,
I hear myself described as 'very active' by a young doctor,
and I hope sincerely that this is a positive statement on my
fitness, rather than an assessment of my disease's progress.
Then the consultant enters and sits, speaking and listening
attentively. A CAT scan and 'cardiograph are needed and
noted, and then it is time to speak of the *treatment*.
I hear that I have a 'narrowed choice' of drugs.
Asking the derivation of the ones prescribed for me,
I learn that they are plant-derived. This seems fitting on a
day that began with gardening, and luminous leaves.
I decide to envisage my tumours as unwanted weeds,
invading me, an otherwise healthy garden, and the chemo-
drugs acting as weedkiller. The image helps.
Finally, I hear about some side effects from this particular
compound. 'You will lose your hair, you will feel sick, and
you will be vulnerable to infection. We will watch that.'
Just facts to take on board, communicated kindly.
The sun continues to shine.

PRAYING

Lord,
I remember my mother could fuss about
nothing, but when it came to bigger things
she took it on the chin and came through.
I feel a bit like that.
I will be bald, and I will possibly feel sick,
though medications will help.
This has a beginning and an ending.
Let me take it with my mother's kind of spirit
and with Your and her, kind of help.
Amen.

Just one word or sentence might be the one that opens the way for your own journey, inwards and onwards.

- 'My own stark realities are/have been ...'
  Finish the sentence and write onwards.

- The effect/your response:

- Your inner and outer resources are:

- The person most supportive at this time is:

- Five keywords for journaling:

Prayer-starter
- Using any medium – paint, markers, crayons, charcoal, pastels, etc. – create your own image of any of the above, and pray from that.

- Insights from prayer:

I will be your God through all your life-time
yes, even when your hair is white with age,
I made you and I will care for you.

Isaiah 46:3–4 Living Bible

15

THE CHALLENGE OF THE JUG

'At your age' is a phrase I have begun to hear frequently in
the hospital where I sit today, waiting for a CAT scan.
I reach to stow away my phone, when suddenly my age
comes against me, because this phone is too new and too
smart and I don't know how to switch it off.
However something else is happening,
which drops that phone right out of my mind.
I am staring directly at the Challenge of the Jug.
Being filled with liquid and having to retain enough for a
CAT scan can be a challenge for oldies. I watch in horror
as a smiling receptionist hands an elderly man a litre jug
of juice and a small clipboard to record the intervals of
emptying it. The same fate awaits me.
Initially, the regular recording of sips distracts me, but as
the time mounts up, I am impelled to abandon both my
seat and the plastic cup, and edge my discomforted way
towards the reception desk. I gesture, without much hope,
towards that closed door with its unisex shapes. 'Oh no,
that's all right! Work away!' Relief! I had only to ask!
Later I lie, gowned and lined, and facing upwards, under
the scanner. Two little red-cheeked emoticons are stuck to
it, showing how to hold ones breath. I want to laugh.
The machine's clicks and rotates, taking me all in. I look up
and think, 'you can see inside me, but right now I can see
inside you, too!'. Soon all is over, and I am elbow-guided
back to reception by a very young man who also shows me
how to manage my phone.
'No problem! I have to do this all the time for my nan.'
(The age groups need each other!).

PRAYING

Lord,
Today I am thanking you
for that part of older age
which is always a learner.
I am thanking you for
all the tiny opportunities
for new knowledge,
even about phones.
I am thanking you too
that my age
has brought me beyond
youthful embarrassments
and I can state my needs,
including bathroom needs.

JOURNAL
For you

Just one word or sentence might be the one that opens the way for your own journey, inwards and onwards.

· 'Age? Let me tell you ...'
Finish the sentence and write onward.

· A family history of genes, siblings and self:

· A list of age-challenges would include:

· A list of age-positives would include:

· A pamphlet for 'Tips for living' in older age:

· Your 'sage-stage' motto:

· Five keywords for journaling:

Prayer-starter
· Ponder a quote of age-stage wisdom. If necessary, amend, adapt, rewrite and pray as your own.

· Insights from prayer:

Let your 'Yes' be yes and your 'No' be no.

James 5:12

16

COMMITTING TO THE PROCESS

A friend's husband has given me a lift to the hospital.
Whilst opening the car door, he says something
particularly true and profound, given that today I will find
out my chemotherapy schedule.
'When we are open, and invited to embrace something,
then we are taken to another level of awareness.'
I climb the stairs, fortified by the thought, and step into
the waiting room. I don't want to read. I want to think.
My turn comes, and the consultant explains everything.
He carefully details my treatment dates, waiting quietly
while I fumble with little pages, inept, and with my head
muddled. I can't get it right. Finally, he takes my pen
and marks each date into my diary himself. In the very
middle of this treatment schedule, beckoning temptingly,
is my long anticipated, already booked Summer holiday.
Through blissful ignorance, I blithely propose that the
holiday might go ahead anyway, despite these carefully
planned, all-encompassing, written-in dates. He looks at
me. Steadily. It's like, 'No way.' He pauses before saying,
kindly but firmly, 'You don't want to compromise the
process.' I take that as a statement. It's simple. It's the
truth. 'I don't want to be stupid,' I say, subsiding. His eyes
tell me that to go breaking this schedule of cycles would
indeed be stupid.

PRAYING

Lord,
Thank you for that.
A part of me has been missing the point.
I have been 'going along with'
all the new information
but today, through a small example,
I realise I haven't yet taken in the whole picture.
A part of me has been standing to one side,
half believing that I can carry on just as usual.
I get it now. I can't.
This is about me, personally,
not anyone else.
It's an invitation
to accept or not accept
in freedom,
to commit to a treatment plan,
trusting and embracing it with awareness.
My true self knew this
So help me live from that true self.
I commit.
Amen.

- 'When we are open, and invited to embrace something, then we are taken to another level of awareness.'
  True or false for you at the moment?

- 'I am making a commitment because ...'
  Finish the sentence and write onwards.

- 'Why I am not making a commitment is because ...'
  Finish the sentence and write onwards.

- The costs (emotional, physical, familial, financial) involved in a current commitment are:

- Compromise, collaboration, co-operation, competition, co-ordination. Choose a word and expand on its meaning and application for you.

- Five keywords for journaling:

Prayer-starter
- Weighing up options through a discernment process. Where is the core peace – in and of God – to be found? Sit with this, and if necessary with a mentor or wise prayer-guide.

- Insights from prayer:

Do not fear, for I am with you; do not be afraid,
for I am your God. I will strengthen you; I will help you.

Isaiah 41:10

17

GATHERING MYSELF TOGETHER

Today I have my first session of chemo. Crazily, I have been cha-cha-cha-ing to early morning music. I believe that I am insuring against the possibility that I might not feel like dancing, later. (Or maybe I will.)

But then I find myself cleaning my teeth for the second time and reluctantly admit that I am feeling vulnerable. Perhaps it's the thought of absorbing something, however beneficial, which I can't pick up off a plate. However, once this is acknowledged, I conjure a lively mental picture of healthy cells mustering for resistance and recovery, and tumour cells falling back, vanquished.

Bus to the hospital, and I join a group of people in the waiting bay. To my inexperienced, furtively room-sweeping eyes, some look rather exhausted. Perhaps this is because it is not yet 8 a.m. Anyway they are talking to one another. They are smiling at me. Understanding.

The waiting area empties and people move on into the treatment ward. Then the friendly receptionist calls my name and nods for me to 'follow the nurse'. But suddenly I don't want to follow anyone. I find I have mutinied. The nurse is already quite far down the hall. I want her here. Now I see why they suggest you 'bring someone with you'. The nurse turns round. She begins to come back. I stand up. I begin to walk. I feel like a frightened puppy.

PRAYING

Lord,
I am asking you to give me courage
and strength to engage with this treatment,
and I ask that every cell will understand
what it is it has to do.
Heart still in mouth, yet involved,
I am tapping into creation
and research, and science
and the mysterious
healing properties of plants and compounds.
I am thankful to you for all of that
and that I am able to be part of it.
I haven't forgotten that so many can't.
I am grateful.

Just one word or sentence might be the one that opens the way for your own journey, inwards and onwards.

· 'What I am fearing in this present situation is ...'
  Finish the sentence and write onward.

· 'My image of myself in this situation is ...'
  Finish the sentence and write onward, or colour and draw.

· A true story of a time of insecurity was:

· A dialogue with a wisdom figure would sound like:

· My coping skills include:

· Five keywords for journaling:

Prayer-starter
· Draw and label your own present 'Support Tree' – those around you physically, or near in spirit, who constitute the roots, the trunk, the branches, the twigs and the individual leaves in support and presence. Pray from an awareness of this.

· Insights from prayer:

May your roots go down deep into the soil of God's marvellous love; and may you be able to feel and understand ... how wide, how long, how deep and how high his love really is; and to experience this.

Ephesians 3:17–18 NRSV

18

FIRST CHEMO DAY

Chemo ward, and 'We love blood here,' says a smiley nurse, 'And we don't worry too much about time.'

Wha-at? Her name is not Alice, but is this Wonderland? Then she explains what she means – 'We need to test your bloods on each visit, and the important thing is, to have everything correlated, so your meds can be made up just right, by our pharmacist. And it might take a while.' Aah ... suddenly I feel good, part of a team. A little cannula is swiftly and painlessly inserted into my forearm near the wrist 'so it isn't disturbed by any elbow activity'. My bloods are taken, and dispatched for testing, and the nurse then reappears with the equivalent of a goody bag. This is promising. She extracts a particularly soft toothbrush, a tube of toothpaste, and a small bottle of mouthwash. Oral hygiene takes on extra importance. 'This helps to prevent infection.' Then she shows me two little round caps. 'For when you lose your hair – you'd be amazed how warm your hair keeps your head.' My thick hair is still strongly attached to my scalp so I nod with agreement rather than experience. My bloods come back, and shortly after I am attached to the stand from which will hang my fluid source of hope. There is an initial 'flush through' and I briefly feel a cold and slightly tingling sensation, which will become familiar. The drops drip rhythmically according to a setting. My second bag drips through and a beeping announces the last moments of countdown. I rouse as a nurse gently removes my canula and strapping. 'See you again soon!' she says with a little wave.

Oh, I'll be back!

PRAYING

Lord,
where I am
on the recliner chair
others have been.
And others will be again.
This is a system
which works well,
and I have become part of it.
I feel both passive and active.
Passive as to the physical procedures,
yet active in the will to embrace this fully.

....

Just one word or sentence might be the one that opens the way for your own journey, inwards and onwards.

· 'The treatment/ procedure which is part of my life at the moment is ...' Finish the sentence and write onward.

· A typical treatment/procedure day looks like:

· Patient or professional? Better or worse?

· Engaging wholeheartedly with treatment and systems means what for you?

· A letter written from you to the professionals involved in your treatment/nursing/life-situation would say:

· Five keywords for journaling:

Prayer-starter
· One thing in detail, from today, for which to be thankful.

· Insights for Prayer:

The Lord is my shepherd – he makes me lie down, he restores my soul.

UCB Psalm 23:2–3

19
NOT QUITE MYSELF

My head feels 'swimmy' and heavy,
like a bottle cap not quite in the correct groove.
A tiredness is creeping up.
I stir awake, feeling slightly sick.
My teeth are chattering.
My heart is thudding.
There's an echo in my head.
After half an hour, as I begin to get up,
all of this subsides, leaving just a tingling in my calves.
Soda water helps.
The reflux, now a knot of discomfort,
sounds its distinctive tummy growl –
growling is an appropriate response
under the circumstances.
I have a multiplication of tablets to take,
and times to take them.
They all have a purpose.
It's all very new and strange,
and the symptoms may be 'nerves',
but whatever,
as my mother might have said
peering at me as a child,
'You're not quite yourself.'
Exactly.

PRAYING

Lord,
I thought I knew my body.
Prided myself on self-awareness,
self-care,
fitness, flexibility.
But now it feels under siege
and is reacting accordingly.
They told me what to expect
and I am being given the means to cope.
No need to panic.
Help me stay steady
and do this right.

Just one word or sentence might be the one that opens the way for your own journey, inwards and onwards.

· 'Not myself' feels like:

· Strategies and remedies and why they have worked:

· Your body's personal letter to you:

· 'The particular things I keep note of in terms of my health are ...' Finish the sentence and write onward.

· Five keywords for journaling:

Prayer-starter
· Taking your time, praying as if within each part of your body in turn.

· Insights from prayer:

From His goodness we have all received, grace upon grace.

John 1:16

20

WARMING UP

Convivial – a warm and genial word, but not overdramatic.
I now experience the chemo ward as convivial. With each
day's visit, I've settled in.
We aren't over-chatty, but we have got to know one
another. The usual social niceties aren't needed.
We by-passed all that. We are down to basics.
Very humanising, very equalising. When you're wired up
to an IV stand, or just lying quietly awaiting good news
about bloods, a smile or an understanding word goes
a long way. The nurses are cheerful and welcome us by
name. Did I say 'us'? Yes, it is an 'us'.
We are all in this together. The atmosphere is warming. As
I say, not dramatic: convivial.
For some time this morning, a nurse has been trying to
entice my veins to release the necessary blood samples.
She enlists the help of a colleague but ... no blood.
Although I am 'a bleeder', I am evidently initially a blood
hoarder. I wish they could say what was once said of a
friend. 'Oh, he's got such lovely veins!'
However, they can't and finally it's 'the wrap'.
My arm is ensconced in the enhanced pillow equivalent of
an electric blanket. I relax and read the paper. Time passes.
This other warmth opens my veins and my lifeblood is
finally released.

PRAYING

Lord,
What opens the veins, opens the heart.
We expand and deliver in warmth.
We are able to give when relaxed
we smile when welcomed.
We feel good when we belong,
help me to be warm
and respond to warmth.

JOURNAL
For you

Just one word or sentence might be the one that opens the way for your own journey, inwards and onwards.

· Memories and associations with the word 'warmth' are:

· Work environments that involve 'out of the box' creative thinking are:

· 'The wrap' – all the associations with that word.

· 'What "closes me up" is …'
  Finish and write on from the sentence.

· Five keywords for journaling:

Prayer-starter
· Light a candle and ponder the mystery and source and symbolism of light, warmth, fire.

· Insights from prayer:

I will instruct you and teach you the way you should go.

Psalm 32:8 NRSV

21

THE CHUCKLING TAXI DRIVER

I have been given the unexpected
but creative gift of taxi money
for these sessions,
so today,
as it is pouring with rain,
I decide to forget the bus
and take a taxi.
The traffic is heavy
and, climbing aboard
as a well-seasoned walker,
I propose for the taxi driver
the route I think
will take us to the hospital
in a flash.
The driver laughs heartily
as he heads off in a completely
different direction.
'When people say to use that street you are saying, I always
smile, because I know that by the time we reach it, you
will be crying. We know. Taxi drivers always know!' He
chuckles with the contentment of sureness. He knows he
is on the right road.

PRAYING

Lord,
thank you for this great example
of self-confidence
and sureness
and humour.
It is a great combination.
This was someone who knew where he was going,
and how to get there.
In my life, let me also
be sure that I know where
I am going and why.
And if I am not sure,
let me have the honesty to admit it,
and be prepared to make time
to stop and review my reasoning,
with you.

JOURNAL
For you

....

Just one word or sentence might be the one that opens the way for your own journey, inwards and onwards.

- Create a timeline of your life's journey so far, noting the significant dates, events, and reasons for remembering these in particular.

- Someone who really made an impression:

- 'My Way' could be summed up in these words:

- 'What gives me happiness about the journey I am on is ...' Finish the sentence and write onward.

- Five keywords for journaling:

Prayer-starter
- Ponder your timeline, and pray from any one moment on it that still holds energy for you – positive or negative. Place it confidently in the space for prayer.

- Insights from prayer:

I have called you by name; you are mine.
... you are precious in my sight,
and honoured, and I love you.

Isaiah 43:1–2

22

MY HAIR'S GONE

My hair has all gone,
exactly as they said it would.
It began with those few stray hairs on the pillow.
Then it all looked noticeably thinner,
and I began to see light through its curly-ness.
Then there were the telltale tufts
in the teeth of my comb
and the tufts began to come away
with the ease of carrots
lifting from the soil. Disconcerting. Uneven.
So it had to be done.
The shave.
My phone holds a picture of before and after.
It was good to have my friend do it. He didn't laugh.
Nor did my neighbours when I asked them
if I had a 'rudimentary' head, maybe like a peanut?
They said, 'No, your head looks pretty normal.'
Then 'Actually, you have quite a good head.'
That's nice. I never knew.
(Funny how we see ourselves –
but then who can see the whole of their own head?)
My other neighbour said, 'It doesn't make any difference.'
And so tonight I realised something:
my hair *is* lost, but something else is found.
A 'this is me, just as I am' candour.
A silent, but immensely deep, loud,
joyful bald shout to the naked universe.

PRAYING

Lord,
I have given my hair a bad press
all my life. Too curly, too thick,
when I wanted straight and sleek.
Well, it's all gone now.
I believe it will return. I trust it will return.
How? Will I have turned grey?
I am finally engaging with loving my hair,
however and whenever it returns, and meanwhile
also loving my not-a-peanut head.

Just one word or sentence might be the one that opens the way for your own journey, inwards and onwards.

· Society's main body messages:

· 'Self-image for me means ...'
  Finish the sentence and write onward.

· A love letter to yourself:

· 'What has affected my body and my feelings ...'
  Finish the sentence and write onward.

· A 'this is truly me' poem:

· 'The most inner liberating experience of my life so far
  has been ...' Finish the sentence and write onward.

· Five keywords for journaling:

Prayer-starter
· Being present to that realness which remains the
  freeing core of being, deeper than shape, size, hair, no
  hair, scars, losses, etc.

· Insights from prayer:

O Give thanks to the Lord, for he is good;
for his steadfast love endures forever.

Psalm 107:1

23

GOOD ENERGY DAY

This is a day of good energy.
It feels like tingles of Life
flickering throughout my body
and re-awakening my brain.
They come every second week,
like waves rising and falling.
This week the rise allows creative cooking
for cousins from 'abroad'
and before that wave moves to crest
and then flow into energy flatness
I will make sure to see friends,
walk to the market,
cook and wash-up.
I will feel I am living well,
without a 2 p.m. nap
or an 8 p.m. bedtime,
– indispensable in the
plug-pulling energy drain of
the Other Days.
Outside there is a toddler,
chattering, running up and down.
I hear her bright little voice
as a voice of growth and renewing life.

PRAYING

Lord,
this is a gratitude day
for the littlest things.
Which today feel like big things.
Thank you for the hours when I have energy
enough for the visitors I can enjoy and eat with.
Chemo is not a blip on my nice smooth life-path.
It IS my path.
All of it.
I feel a sense of peace.
Just welling up.
Like quiet joy.

JOURNAL
For you

....

Just one word or sentence might be the one that opens the way for your own journey, inwards and onwards.

- 'A day of good energy for me is ...'
  Finish the sentence and write onwards.

- Your daily gratitude journal. Write today's entry.

- 'One of the best celebrations ever, was ...'

- 'Energy boosts' come from:

- Five keywords for journaling:

Prayer-starter
- Your own psalm of awareness/thanksgiving:

- Prayer for energetic people in your family or circle:

- Insights from prayer:

My grace is sufficient for you. For power is made perfect in weakness ... the power of Christ may dwell in me.

2 Cor 12:9–10

24

TINY TRIUMPHS

Not so many years ago,
I remember saying to a friend,
'I'm not sure I know what tired feels like.'
Well, on a non-energy day,
I could eat those words.
(If I felt able to eat.)
Did I ever notice the twenty steps down to my front door?
Never mind that, I can't even walk up my house stairs.
The idle bannister is now my crutch
and crawling upwards, is a viable option.
Triumph is reaching the top,
but not a triumph to be repeated too often.
I leave a day's detritus on the lowest step.
Morning's energy spurt runs out
and folds me onto the sofa
– an interim bed. I doze,
but the tiredness feels limitless.
My body is a sack of sand.

PRAYING

Lord,
I made it!
No hubris, just glad.
Glad I woke up.
Glad for my sofa.
Glad for one more day down
until next week, when I trust
I will feel that faint stirring
in my deepest core.
Thank you for the gift of life,
and I pray for an energy field
that will expand again, to include
the possibility of stairs.

. . . .

Just one word or sentence might be the one that opens the way for your own journey, inwards and onwards.

- 'I recognise when energy is running low, because ...'
  Finish the sentence and write onwards.

- The challenges when energies run low are:

- 'Today the challenge was ...'
  Finish the sentence and write onward.

- Small steps, small triumphs:

- 'The person whose life inspires me is ...'
  Finish the sentence and write onward.

- Five keywords for journaling:

Prayer-starter
- When you can't do anything else, then simply 'become like the earth, receiving the sun.' (Anthony Bloom)

- Insights from prayer:

Love is very patient and kind.

1 Cor 13:4 Living Bible.

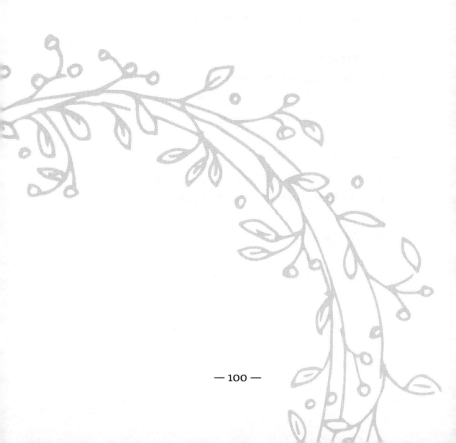

25

COUGHS AND KINDNESS

I don't have leprosy but today I felt like a leper.
With my chemo-weakened immune system,
I have caught a 'bug'
which is now a full-blown rasping chest-infection.
I am in the hospital
for a mid-treatment checkup
and though full,
the waiting room is very very quiet.
No one is talking.
Is anyone breathing?
I breathe. *Wheeze. Wheeze* ...
Cough.
Cough! It's a throat strangler with a tickle
COUGH! A tear-jerker.
N.B. No-one in here needs an infection.
Their immune systems are weaker too.
They know this. Yet no-one turns away.
No-one leaves the room.
Instead, someone stretches out
to offer a paper cup of water.
'It's very warm out there.'
Another proffers a sweet.
They are so forgiving.
So kind.
'Was that you coughing out there?' asks my oncologist,
reaching for a prescription pad.

PRAYING

Lord,
here's my thinking.
There are places where
it is appropriate to blend in.
A hospital waiting room
is one of them.
You take your allotted place,
and, quietly patient,
in a suspended time-warp,
you passively wait your turn.
No-one expects to jump the queue
or push for any favours.
But today, noisily, and contagiously,
I was not blending in.
In fact, I was 'disturbing the peace'.
Yet all I received was kindness.

Just one word or sentence might be the one that opens the way for your own journey, inwards and onwards.

· A time you have felt like a 'nuisance' or, as you might tell yourself, 'a burden':

· Tell the story from your point of view, and then from the other person's point of view.

· 'Spontaneous moments of kindness ...'
Recall a moment of kindness in your life.

· 'The last time I sat in a doctor's waiting room ...'
Finish the sentence and write onwards as a funny story.

· Five keywords for journaling:

Prayer-starter
· Pray for carers, and those you know, in need of special care at home.

· Insights from prayer:

When you pass through the waters,
I will be with you.
and through rivers, they shall not overwhelm you
when you walk through fire, you shall not be burned
and the flame shall not consume you.
For I am the Lord your God.

Isaiah 43:2–3.

26

HONESTLY

Seriously.
Truthfully.
Honestly.
Today, I am struggling.
I feel I smell different.
My scalp is tingling.
My jaw is stiff, and it is like
I can't open my mouth wide any more.
Not that I want to.
Every bite tastes like bland blanket.
Only milk has any taste, and that
seems sugary-sweet. Weird.
Even my nails have discoloured.
No lashes or eyebrows
so mine is the 'pink-eyed rabbit' look.
(That plus my usual Bugs Bunny teeth!)
I hear this will all pass, but
today feels like the longest day.
I couldn't even unscrew the milk carton
(who can?) and I still have that chest infection.

PRAYING

'This too shall pass'
I always liked that phrase.
Comforting.
So Lord, reassure me that
this too shall pass,
as I experience my body as never before.
Yes, things will change,
as they already have.
I am adapting, living
just half a day at a time.
And in today's first half
I am telling you,
I feel weak.
And I really don't like it.
Who would?

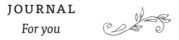

. . . .

Just one word or sentence might be the one that opens the way for your own journey, inwards and onwards.

·   'Today I am struggling because ...'
Finish the sentence and write onwards.

·   The taste-bud story:

·   Favourite summer menus:

·   'This too shall pass'

·   Five keywords for journaling:

Prayer-starter
·   Jesus says, 'Come as you are ...'

·   Insights from prayer:

To make an apt answer is a joy to anyone!
And a word in season, how good it is!

Proverbs 15:23

27

NO VOICE

The chest infection is receding,
but my voice has disappeared.
So my best effort is a chesty squeak.
It is not possible to breathe
and talk at the same time.
I want to talk, but I have to gasp,
which makes my friends also gasp
(especially on the phone).
'You sound terrible!'
I don't actually feel terrible,
just mute.
A second course of antibiotics
has struggled for supremacy but failed,
and now it's the turn of the steroid and the inhaler.
'Something really stuck down there,' says my GP.
(Paradoxically, the chemo is almost a breeze by
comparison. Everything is relative.)

PRAYING

Lord,
This 'losing my voice'
makes me aware
of the times
when I have a voice
and could speak
but fail to speak.
Out of – preferring to please?
Laziness? Can't be bothered?
Even some fear of consequence?
But then there are the times
in my interests of 'truth' at all costs,
when I do claim to 'say it as it is!'
But what about the hearer?
It's a fine line. What is truth?
This enforced silence
is a private little seminar on
stepping back into mindfulness.
Choosing words with more thoughtful care,
honouring words, savouring words –
and Lord, when I find I have run out of words
and preferably before,
let me listen out for yours.

Just one word or sentence might be the one that opens the way for your own journey, inwards and onwards.

· 'What I really want to say is ...'
Finish this sentence and write onwards.

· 'I have often regretted my speech, but never my silence' (Publius Syrus, 85-43 BC). You?

· Are you a talker or a listener?

· 'Mindfulness' of the tongue is:

· 'Everything is relative' ... in your situation meaning what?

· Five keywords for journaling:

Prayer-starter
· What is it that you don't bring into prayer? What is it that you don't say? Why not?

· Insights from prayer:

Come to me, all you that are weary and are carrying heavy burdens, and I will give you rest.

Matthew 11:28

28

ACCEPTING MY LIMITS

There has been
an army of tiny elves
wielding miniature pickaxes,
and jabbing
at the joints of my legs and feet.
So random.
So sharp.
I'm twitching
and twitchy.
Saying 'ouch!'
and walking as if two inches above the ground.
'Platform feet!'
Then, I remember.
The hospital said it clearly.
'Tell us! Give feedback!'
No need for stoics.
I fed back.
The dose is reduced.
Wonderful!
No more elves.
No more miniature hammers.
I am glad I said it.

PRAYING

Lord,
help me to be aware
and respectful of my limits,
acknowledging when I have reached
my threshold
and not try and 'brave it out'
for no good reason,
when a word
in the right place
can change things
for the better
and
continue the process
of healing.

Just one word or sentence might be the one that opens the way for your own journey, inwards and onwards.

· 'Anyone who is not a stoic is a whinger.'
Agree or disagree?

· 'I first noticed my limitations when ...'
Finish the sentence and write onwards.

· 'A situation that is testing me is ...'
Finish the sentence and write onwards.

· What to say, who to tell, how to say it: these are the questions. What are the answers?

· Five keywords for journaling:

Prayer-starter
· Ponder the Station of the Cross where Simon of Cyrene shoulders the cross of Jesus, or read the account of this in Luke 23:26.

· Insights from prayer:

Be still, and know, that I am God.

Psalm 46:10 NRSV

29

JUST; NOW

For many years it has been,
'Well, I really did the garden for my mum.
I'd never have time to sit in it myself'
True or false,
NOW, I do.
Today (as always), sun touched and warmed my cheek
But TODAY, I knew it.
Felt grateful.
Less energy is loss, but consciousness is the gain.
Moving more slowly.
I have time to notice.
Clouds are not white, but pearl.
Leaves are not green
but have turned rusty saffron.
My beans are fibrous pods by now
dangling above tomatoes which have burst,
beyond shininess, onto the messy gravel.
Tits clinging to the nut nets
dare dining in my presence.
They are safe, and I feel safe.
I am content with whatever time I have left.
I am not ambitious to do anything,
or be anything, beyond what I am,
Now.
Today I felt one with Creation.

PRAYING

Lord,
Whatever happens out of this
Whether I die or whether I live
Let me remember the thoughts of today
That I am content with who I am
And that time is a gift in which to receive.
If later on I am to give again,
then let it be
out of a place of enrichment
for I have met the Source,
newly, and specially
in Now.

Just one word or sentence might be the one that opens the way for your own journey, inwards and onwards.

- Write a body-mind relaxation meditation.

- 'Clouds' – Your poem

- 'Now' – Your poem

- Observe birds, fish, or a pet, and write about what you notice.

- Your real (or imagined) garden looks like:

- What brings you contentment? Describe.

- 'The time of my life is ...'
  Finish the sentence and write onwards.

- Five keywords for journaling:

Prayer-starter
- Observing something from the garden or field, or creating something from natural materials, then with mindful awareness enter into contemplative silence.

- Insights from prayer:

AUTUMN

God has given each of you some special abilities; be sure
to use them to help each other, passing onto others God's
many kinds of blessings.

1 Peter 4:10

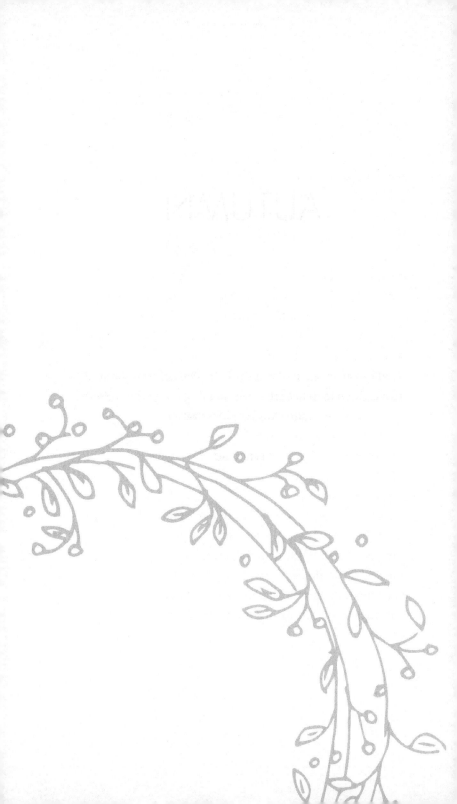

30

ALL TOGETHER BEFORE
THE HOSPITAL GATE

I used to think that being stuck in a lift
would be the ultimate scenario
of unlikely fellowship.
But when I once was, no one spoke at all.
My current experience of fellowship
is not like that.
We are pedestrians, and we are all talking,
united in desire to reach the hospital gates.
Autumn rain is slashing sideways,
and we are marooned on a small cement island
between six lanes of traffic,
at a halfway crossing-point,
with two feeder lanes spurting cars
into the roaring mainstream, either side of us.
It feels seriously dangerous.
The question, 'Why did the chicken cross the road'
is easily answered here.
Every few seconds,
a few experienced (or reckless) individuals
break free from the soaked crush of bodies
and the slowest of traffic-light cycles,
and scuttle perilously to the hospital gates.
The remainder watch helplessly and wonder,
'Did anyone ever think of a footbridge?'

PRAYING

Lord,
Today, a routine appointment morning,
I felt fellowship
with those
who, for whatever reason,
did not enter the hospital
in relative comfort and dryness.
Whatever is waiting for them once inside,
it hurts that that sick-looking man
had to stand too long in the chilling rain,
or that child with her mother.
The quiet young man in the wheelchair –
I have met him before. With his brother.
And I feel especially close to the older people,
hatted and gloved even now,
who, like myself,
are simply unable to flee
before the 'green man' appears,
affording us safe passage.
'But what can we do?' they say.
That's my question.
I need to find an answer.

Just one word or sentence might be the one that opens the way for your own journey, inwards and onwards.

- 'A present situation that stirs me enough to want to complain, protest, or write about it is ...'
  Finish this sentence and write onward.

- Is the above affecting you or others, or both? Describe.

- The values that really matter:

- Your petition:

- Five keywords for journaling:

Prayer-starter
- Pray for the people affected by the matter at hand. Ask to know your part in this, how not to hinder, how to help.

- Insights from prayer:

Trust in the Lord with all your heart, and lean not on your own understanding."

Proverbs 3:5-6

31

SURGICAL STEPS

The months have passed
the lump has shrunk
and now what needs to go, will go.
The problem seems to be more under the breast
than right in the breast.
Does that give me options?
Another mammogram
and a visit to the awesomely-named
'Nuclear Medicine' centre.
'A little bit of a sting,' they tell me considerately,
as isotopic injections pierce the skin
but I find myself thinking,
'when you've had upper-lip electrolysis,
stinging is a relative term.'
Then, the last stage of preparation
finds me marked with a marker;
A neat blue arrow drawn on my skin
indicates clearly which breast to target.
So, marked, tagged and labelled,
I am an alert parcel, ready to be sent through.
I am paused in the pre-op bay,
my wrist encircled with proof of identity,
while a third nurse verifies that this is really me.
'We want to make sure we have the correct patient.'
Proper order. This is good.

PRAYING

Lord,
I remember an engineer once telling me,
'It's all about preparation.'
I was impatient, had a project
and was not keen to wait.
But he stood his ground,
and the work was the better for it.
Today I'm being 'prepped' for an operation.
But truly another preparation
has been happening for months.
A preparation beyond skin,
a preparation in patience,
a preparation in perspective,
and a preparation in perception.
Thank you for this time.

JOURNAL
For you

Just one word or sentence might be the one that opens the way for your own journey, inwards and onwards.

- 'Ready!' You are being prepared for what? And you feel? The time of preparation has lasted how long? Write your story.

- 'The insights I have gained from a time of extended preparation are ...' Finish the sentence and write onwards.

- 'Internal preparation is about ...' Finish the sentence and write onwards.

- 'We want to make sure we have the correct person.' How do you respond to this sentence? What labels would you attach to yourself to identify you as you?

- Write a paragraph on patience, perspective or perception.

- Five keywords for journaling:

Prayer-starter
- Choose your own identifying tag or 'label' and pray from there. Is this the name God knows you by too?

- Insights from prayer:

I was helpless in the hands of God. And when he said to me, 'Go out into the valley, and I will talk to you there,' I arose and went, and Oh! I saw the glory of the Lord.

Ezekiel 4:22

32

ON THE OPERATING TABLE

The operating theatre.
'I am in your hands!'
I shuffle onto, and then lie down on,
the operating table.
The IV line is inserted into my hand,
and chattily, my blood-pressure is checked:
'For someone about to have an operation,
that is very good!'
So chat must have worked!
The atmosphere is genial.
The Team, standing in a half-circle,
are gowned and gloved
and looking ready.
I am gowned.
Am I ready?
It is noonday-bright.
There is that circular light,
familiar from TV, positioned above my head.
I guess it will 'come on' after I 'go out!'
This thought triggers a final grab at tangible reality.
'What is the wattage of that lamp?'
An irrelevant question.
I could not have interpreted the answer,
even if they had told me,
which they might have done,
only the anaesthetic is taking over,
and the ceiling is starting to sway.

PRAYING

Lord,
anaesthesia always feels
like an ultimate surrender
It is a sensation that I actually like,
because it is more than sensation.
It is an attitude
of trust and hope.
Not in oblivion
but in destination.

JOURNAL
For you

. . . .

Just one word or sentence might be the one that opens the way for your own journey, inwards and onwards.

- 'For me, an operation means ...'
  Finish the sentence and write onwards.

- 'The thing I really remember ...'
  Write the story

- For you, the phrase 'surrender to the process', means:

- Your psalm/prayer/song/poem of hope and trust:

- Five keywords for journaling:

Prayer-starter
- Your own prayer of surrender.

- Insights from prayer:

Do not worry, saying, 'What will we eat?' or 'What will we drink?' or 'What will we wear?' ... Your heavenly Father knows that you need all these things.

Matt 6:31, 34. NRSV

33

HOSPITAL TOAST

I am in the ward,
post-op
and it's 6 p.m. and time for supper.
I hear the promising clatter of trays
and could be hungry.
The crispy chicken *vol-au-vent*
on the table beside me
looks tempting.
As I ponder the possibilities,
my mind is made up for me.
'You won't be wanting that,
I'll get you some toast.'
Kindly meant, professionally experienced,
and maybe I was being saved from myself.
I will never know.
Hospital toast after fasting
tastes like Heaven.

PRAYING

Lord,
I had to see the humour in this.
How precious I can be
in a restaurant.
Just so, and some of that
and none of this,
all just so it adds up to perfect.
And that vol-au-vent looked perfect
but it wasn't for me, after all.
Let it go.
Life goes on.

JOURNAL
For you

. . . .

Just one word or sentence might be the one that opens the way for your own journey, inwards and onwards.

·   'My favourite comfort food is ...'
    Finish the sentence and write onwards.

·   The incident that brought you to a moment of insight:

·   'Precious' behaviours around food or drink:

·   Write a 'mindful eating' exercise.

·   'Taken away' or let-go?

·   Five keywords for journaling:

Prayer-starter
·   Making peace with what is, rather than what is not.

·   Insights from prayer:

Pleasant words are like a honeycomb,
sweetness to the soul and health to the body.

Proverbs 16:24

34

WARD WIT

'City are away to Spurs on Saturday!'
'Relegation!'
'Haven't beaten Arsenal!'
'Have to have about twelve games
before you'd get a handle on it!'
The debate is fierce, and the two speakers,
friends of course,
are obviously known to the ward,
as 'characters'.
They are enjoying themselves enormously.
I doze, in a dreamy post-operative fog,
letting the cheer lap over me.
A nurse passes by.
One of the characters calls out,
'I'll have a Guinness if you're ordering!'
'Powers for me!'
And so it goes.
A moment's Star turn of entertainment.

PRAYING

Lord,
it did my heart good
to inadvertently share
in such ease.
A self-ease
that beamed around the room
and included anyone
within earshot
into its own
playful delight.

JOURNAL
For you

....

Just one word or sentence might be the one that opens the way for your own journey, inwards and onwards.

· The answer to the question, 'How are you getting along today?' is:

· The sporting/musical/social 'thing' that really gets me talking is:

· 'The people who brighten my day are ...'
Finish the sentence and write onwards.

· The 'Character' – Describe.

· Five keywords for journaling:

Prayer-starter
· Remembering those who can make you laugh.

· Insights from prayer:

Take delight in honouring each other.

Romans 12:10b, Living Bible

35

YOUR PRESENCE IS ENOUGH

It is discharge day.
'Morning! Get your things together!
You're off to the discharge room, and
they serve hot breakfasts there.'
'Really?' innate greediness pricks up my ears.
'No, just kidding!'
She brings me to the discharge bay.
Showered and fed,
we 'leavers' sit quietly
against the walls,
awaiting collection.
Thinking our thoughts.
A frail old man is gesturing
to one of the young staff.
It is hard for him to speak clearly, but he manages it.
'I want to give you something to say thank you.'
She's at least sixty years younger than he,
perhaps a nursing assistant.
She pats his hand, sits down beside him,
smiling but earnest.
Then, looking into his eyes, ensuring he can hear,
'Your presence is enough!' she says.

PRAYING

Lord,
That last sentence said it all.
Thank you.
Amen

JOURNAL
For you

....

Just one word or sentence might be the one that opens the way for your own journey, inwards and onwards.

- 'Your presence is enough' To whom could you say these words?

- 'Time to go!' Discharge and collection.

- 'The words that make my ears prick-up are ...'
  Finish the sentence and write onwards.

- The word 'Presence' applies to:

- 'The ways I like to show appreciation are ...'
  Finish the sentence and write onwards.

- Five keywords for journaling:

Prayer-starter
- Create a setting which reminds you of God's presence.

- Insights for prayer:

How precious it is, Lord, to realise that you are thinking about me constantly. I can't even count how many times a day your thoughts turn towards me. And when I wake in the morning, you are still thinking about me.

Psalm 139:17–18

36

R & R & R, AND R

'You might miss the hospital,'
they told me, 'some people do'.
Would I have believed that before this all began?
Probably not.
Now I do.
And a friend, thinking back to her own experience,
remembers, 'It was like a weekly club,
supporting one another. The 'Bravery club!''
Treatment was camaraderie,
catching up.
Time and texts as well as toxins.
Of course one could miss it.
Live well, Rest, Relax and Recuperation,
that is the recommendation,
to which I am adding one more.
'Reflection'.
'Reflect upon your many blessings, of which all
have many ... Not on your past misfortunes,
of which all have some' (Charles Dickens,
in his Christmas writings).
I will use this season to reflect on many blessings.
Readying now for radium.

PRAYING

Lord,
'Counting blessings'
should be a lifetime's work
not a passing phrase.
I thank you for many
and the many in any misfortune.
Reflection tells me where I have come from,
and where I am.
I may not know what's next,
but I know what is Now.
That knowledge is relaxing.
That knowledge allows choices.
Amen

Just one word or sentence might be the one that opens the
way for your own journey, inwards and onwards.

- The season of life you are in? Spring, Summer, Autumn,
  Winter. Image this in colour, prose, prayer, poetry, etc.

- 'Rest, relax, recuperate, and ...'
  Finish the sentence and write onwards.

- Favourite club:

- A significant blessing from this time:

- Five keywords for journaling:

Prayer-starter
- 'Counting blessings' – on paper, pausing to pray with
  each one.

- Insights from prayer:

Wisdom and good judgement live together, for wisdom knows where to discover knowledge and understanding.

Proverbs 8:12

37
MY BODY KNOWS

'Listen to your body' is a recommendation
I have been proffering professionally,
for years.
Now I am applying it to myself.
After all these years together,
what does my body
expect me to know about it already?
It is freshest in the morning;
no morning time is too early.
By contrast, nightfall elicits close-down;
not an owl.
And how does my body recover?
It soothes by silence,
recovering health in cave-like stillness.
Recovering health in Now.
No questing or websites or TV or cures.
These jangle with options, too many words.
For if you're 'in treatment'
every stranger,
and even someone closer,
has a story.
Everyone has The Way.
For you.
They surely mean well,
but ultimately
it has to be 'Listen to your own body.'

PRAYING

Lord,
Help me to honour the wisdom
that you have embedded in my being,
that tells me instinctively
'Thus and no further
or This and not that.'
Let me not be sucked from my centre
by any enthusiasm which is not part of my own story.
I shall know which is which, by the vibration of energy
that tells me when I have over-reached,
taken an unnecessary detour
and my physical well is dry.

. . . .

Just one word or sentence might be the one that opens the way for your own journey, inwards and onwards.

- What does your body want to tell you about itself?

- Owl or a lark? Extrovert or introvert? Vegan or carnivore? Does it matter?

- 'The things that suck me out of my centre are …' Finish the sentence and write onwards.

- 'Thanks, but no thanks.' Write a story.

- A personal healing prescription for yourself:

- Five keywords for journaling:

Prayer-starter
- Speak the truth with love. Speak with the Lord from your truest self: who you are, how you are, what you need and what others need. Speak to others with that same voice.

- Insights from prayer:

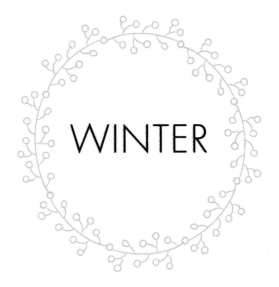

WINTER

Let the Lord ... show us where we should go,
and what we should do ...

Jer 42:3

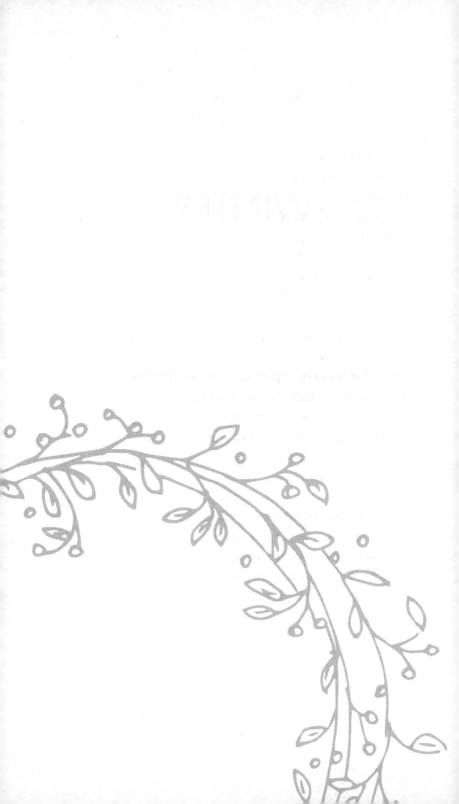

38

RADIOTHERAPY

Every day!
Radiotherapy every day?
My eyes are goggling!
I have been living
on spacious weekly cycles
for nearly a year now
and thinking of *daily* cycles
tightens time into a concertina.
(Why did I have the idea that
all questions were over?)
Well, I obviously didn't think
much at all. But now I am,
and only one question pops up.
'Will I be sunburnt?'
Pale-skinned and with a hat-obsessed past
in African sunshine,
I need to be reassured,
and comprehensively, I am reassured.
The treatment itself is programmed and painless.
The skin is (obviously) monitored daily.
There are proven ways to protect it.
I am especially happy to receive
a methodical list of do's and don't's –
my pro-active involvement in skin-care management.

PRAYING

Lord,
When it was chemo,
I was thinking
of what was happening inside,
now
I am thinking
of what will be happening outside.
Now,
it is about surrendering
to the process;
knowing that it is a process
and that there are stages,
and these are
calibrated,
monitored,
managed
and expected.
Let me embrace each stage as it comes.

JOURNAL
For you

Just one word or sentence might be the one that opens the way for your own journey, inwards and onwards.

- 'Some new information into my life is ...'
  Write this as a letter.

- 'My way of taking in new information is ...'
  Finish the sentence and write onwards.

- An anxious thought around this involves:

- Reassurance around this involves:

- Being pro-active around this involves:

- Five keywords for journaling:

Prayer-starter
- Place a small 'star' sticker on a few ordinary household objects, and each time you notice the sticker, pause and remind yourself, 'You Lord, are my refuge and strength.'

- Insights from prayer:

Lord, you have been our dwelling place in all generations.
Before the mountains were brought forth or ever you had
formed the earth and the world
From everlasting to everlasting, you are God.

Psalm 90:1–2

39

BREATHING NORMALLY

Oh, hello, another blue gown! I had forgotten.
This time, I get to keep it for the entire series of
treatments. That's nice. A memento.
When I am called and enter a treatment room,
I see a giant UFO – surely at the pinnacle of modern
technology.
The radiotherapist helps me onto the treatment table.
My arms are positioned in moulded arm-rests,
and my feet are comfortably supported.
Then my torso is juggled minutely and precisely into place.
The therapists murmur, 'Don't help,'
while rapidly reading out measurements to each other.
This is a swift but concentrated set-up,
and they applaud the machine's accuracy
with satisfied exclamations and cries of 'Excellent!'
This is a good word,
wherever applied, and I find it extremely cheering.
The staff depart to the monitoring kiosk,
instructing me to 'breathe normally'.
Then, with its own in-breath, one of power,
the machine gets down to work.
I feel nothing, only that my solid-enough body
feels strangely slight and soft
by comparison with the shiny sphere of steel
and white plastic that swivels and rotates above me.
Time stands still
until a re-opening door and a bright young voice
announcing, 'All done!' brings me back.

PRAYING
New normal

Lord,
This is about co-operation
with a machine.
I am positioned in the most perfect way
for it to perform exactly and accurately.
I don't have to understand.
I don't have to speak.
I don't have to adjust my body.
I only need to be still.
This is just one more new normal.

Just one word or sentence might be the one that opens the way for your own journey, inwards and onwards.

· New procedures, new skills.

· Monster machines like UFOs.

· 'Co-operating' with the above, either through necessity or practicality, feels like ...

· 'Professionals working for me, and with me, as a team ...' Finish the sentence and write onwards.

· Five keywords for journaling:

Prayer-starter
· Breathe awareness – your body receiving and using oxygen. Breathe the air as God's gift.

· Insights from prayer:

I will give you treasures hidden in the darkness secret riches; and you will know that I am doing this – I the Lord … the one who calls you by your name.

Isaiah 45:3

40
ROUTINES

Ha! Just when I think
I enjoy routine,
I am finding myself
restless with the absolute
necessity of caring for these few inches of skin.
I am sure there is a lesson here, as I
soak gauze with saline, sprinkle with salt,
lather skin with cream, spread cooling gel.
Certainly there is no cracking,
and though red, the skin doesn't hurt.
Attentive looks each day
are accompanied by smiles and a
'Carry on doing what you are' instruction.
So why am I restive with a routine that works?
I have been methodical for months:
pills and potions, rests and routines,
so what's new? Am I just finally bored?
Hardly, the last time I felt bored,
I was about 8 years old.
Why so impatient then?
Am I expecting my body to look after itself?
No, on reflection, this is not boredom,
or impatience.
It is the restiveness of returning life
running riot in muscles and tissues
and re-awakening will.

PRAYING

Yes Lord,
This is life responding to Life.
I am sensing a change of pace in myself,
and I want to move on,
immediately.
Tiredness is no longer holding me back.
If I sleep early and exercise a little,
I am not even tired.
But, as a wise old man used to say,
'Don't run ahead of the Spirit.'
Which right now means
minding that skin.
Do it right,
finish with focus.

....

Just one word or sentence might be the one that opens the way for your own journey, inwards and onwards.

- Your present necessary 'routines':

- Bored, boring, restless, or restive? Write the poem.

- Cared for, or caring for?

- The pros and cons of routines are:

- 'Change of pace, for me, means ...'
  Finish the sentence and write onwards.

- Five keywords for journaling:

Prayer-starter
- 'Don't run ahead of the Spirit.' Ponder, listening for a response.

- Insights from prayer:

Now there was a great wind, so strong that it was splitting mountains and breaking rocks in pieces before the Lord, but the Lord was not in the wind; and after the wind an earthquake, but the Lord was not in the earthquake; and after the earthquake a fire, but the Lord was not in the fire; and after the fire a sound of sheer silence. When Elijah heard it, he wrapped his face in his mantle and went out and stood at the entrance of the cave. Then there came a voice to him that said, 'What are you doing here, Elijah?'

1 Kings 19:11–13

41

PILGRIMAGE

As they continued, these daily sessions
have taken on an aspect of pilgrimage.
It starts with my intention.
I walk to the hospital, different roads,
building stamina bit by bit.
First it was a bus with a short walk.
Then it became a short bus and a longer walk.
Now it is all walk.
Into the radiotherapy unit, then scan
the little appointment book
which cleverly tells the desk, 'She's arrived.'
A ritual drink of water from the gurgling cooler
and I prepare to be a pilgrim proper.
Lying immobile,
alone with the unknown,
for the length of a mindfulness meditation
is an opportunity.
Surrounded by the circling scanner,
I close my eyes and enter into interior silence.
Family members and also friends appear,
paused, one by one, in my mind's eye.
I entrust each one and their particular situation,
to God – my, and their,
surrounding Light.

PRAYING

Lord,
This time of meditation
is precious.
My mind is quiet from the walk.
My body rests. It is not uncomfortable.
I can lie, arms above head,
and offer all out of my hands,
into your hands.
All who come to mind today
for you to take, hold, and heal, and companion,
as you do me. Amen.

JOURNAL
For you

Just one word or sentence might be the one that opens the way for your own journey, inwards and onwards.

- 'When I think of "pilgrimage" …'
  Finish the sentence and write onwards.

- Your personal pilgrimage(s):

- The way to quiet mindfulness:

- My own 'sacred space'.

- Five keywords for journaling:

Prayer-starter
- Holding in God's love and surrounding light, all those you want to remember and pray for.

- Insights from prayer:

SPRING

God lifted me out of the bog and the mire
... and steadied me as I walked along ...
He has given me a new song to sing ...

Psalm 40:2ff, Living Bible

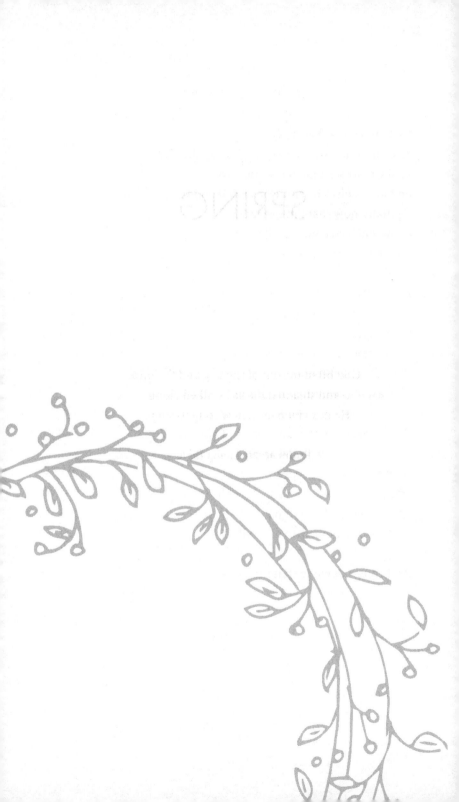

42

THE CIRCLE TURNS

'Only ten more days to go.'
The radiotherapy nurse counts down the days,
as she marks a date in my notebook
and looks with the smile of shared good news.
'Actually, now that I'm used to it,
I have enjoyed coming. I'll miss it.'
She seems amused when I say that.
'Really?'
But it's true.
It has been a sacred time.
It has all been a sacred time.
I remember Viktor Frankl's words:
'There is one freedom.
The last of the human freedoms –
to choose ones's attitude
in whatever circumstance we find ourselves.'
This tells me how to live well.
Now and into my future.
And having lived well, whenever life ends,
I have hope and belief that
I will also be helped to die well.
Yes.
It all comes down to that first 'yes'.

PRAYING

Lord,
Cancer circled through
its own seasons, as well as
Spring, Summer, Autumn, Winter
and into another Spring.
Today it is that season of Spring
which is reflected in myself.
My senses sniff, touch, taste, hear, and see
(for example)
baby blue-tits flying in a feathery frenzy around my
nut-feeder,
life pulsing through the fibres of a branch of buds
on my one apple tree,
and the sky tossing aside its forever blanket,
and turning, for ten minutes,
Mediterranean blue.
This delights me!
But truthfully,
there has been delight in every season.
Every season having its chore and its chance.
I wanted, and want, to choose the chance.

JOURNAL
For you

. . . .

Just one word or sentence might be the one that opens the way for your own journey, inwards and onwards.

· 'Standing on the threshold ...'

· 'Chore, or chance'

· 'For all that has been, thanks. For all that shall be, yes.'
  (Dag Hammarskjold) Write your response as a conversation.

· '"Yes" for me, means ...'
  Finish the sentence and write onward, forever.

· Five keywords for journaling

Prayer-starter
· Experience your own season, own it, and pray with a heart open to receiving the fruits of that season, uniquely for you.

· Insights from Prayer:

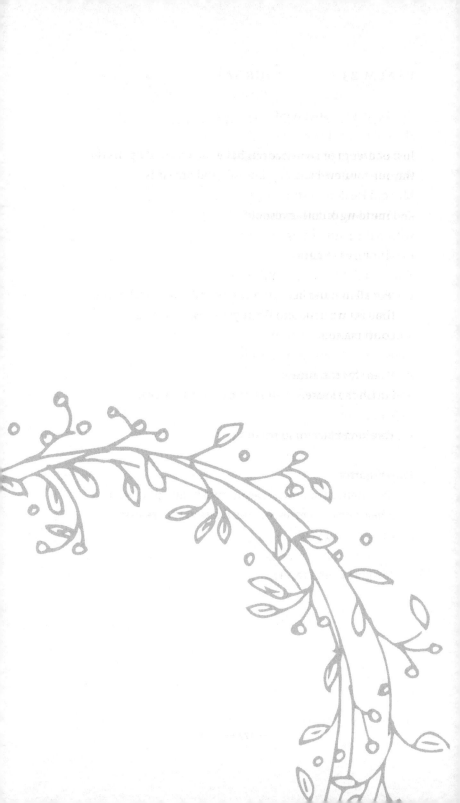

PSALM 23

The Lord is my shepherd, I'll not want
He makes me down to lie.
In pastures green, He leadeth me
the quiet waters by.
My soul He doth restore again
and me to walk doth make
within the paths, of righteousness
e'en for his own namesake.
Yea though I walk in death's dark vale
yet will I fear none ill
for thou art with me and thy rod
and staff me comfort still
Goodness and mercy all my life
shall surely follow me
and in God's House
forever more
my dwelling place shall be.

– Crimmond

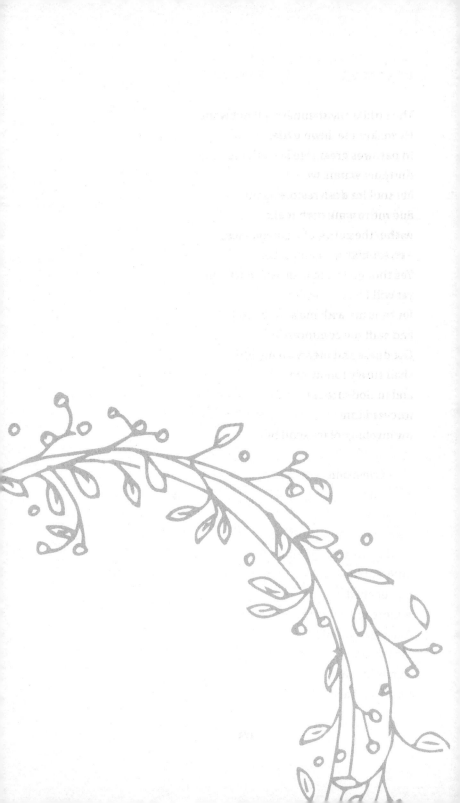

AFTERWORD

My birthday is in July.
As we used to, people have asked
'What's your star sign?'
And I always answered
lightly, 'I'm a July Cancer'
But with an inner wince
At the (then)
'taboo word.'
Cancer.
cancer.
There is no taboo now.
I am still 'a July Cancer'
The cancer aspect I leave to God.
I was treated well.
I remember many friends and acquaintances
who had cancer, but for whom treatment
leading to cure or remission
was not possible.
They live a different Life, now.
For so many others,
like myself,
there has been treatment.
Leading to another kind of
different life.
A deepened life,
A more reflective life
A more mindful life.
Most of all,
a grateful life,
for all, and also

for all who work
the punishing long clinical hours
that we observed and benefitted from.
Consultants, surgeons, doctors,
nurses, therapists.
On them,
many blessings..